GET YOUR WALK ON
Go from 2,000 to 10,000 Steps in 8 Weeks

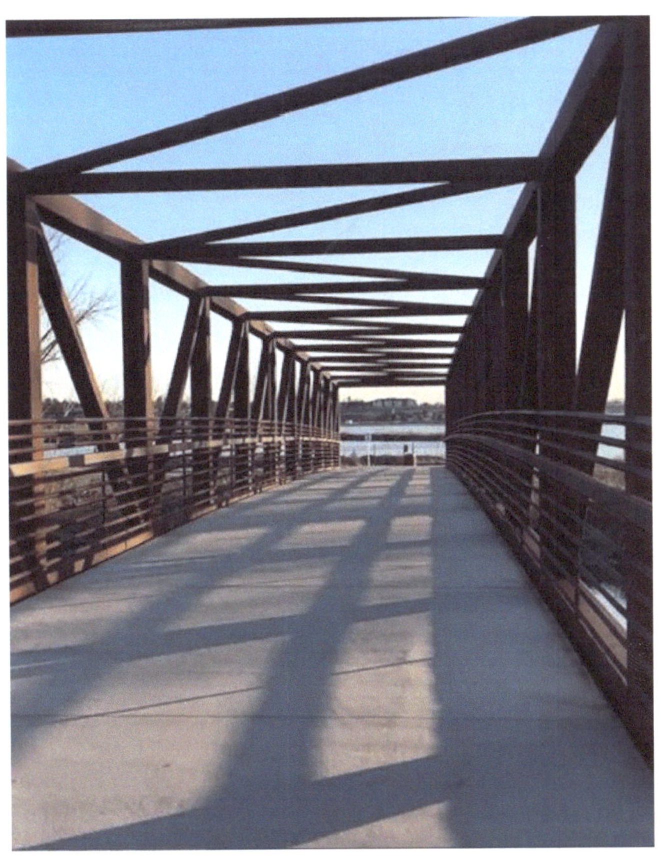

Jeanette R. Harrison, MPH

GET YOUR WALK ON

Go from 2,000 to 10,000 Steps in 8 Weeks

by

Jeanette R. Harrison, MPH

Table of Contents

Foreword

I started filming walking videos for the Billion Steps Challenge in January 2020. Then, COVID hit, and my walking videos became about encouraging other people to get outside, how the diffusion of molecules made the disease less likely to spread, how being outside boosted your immune response, and also increased vitamin D production. My walking videos became about my health and encouraging others to be outside because "outside was okay." If you check out [How Healthcare Works on Instagram](#) or the [How Healthcare Works YouTube channel](#), you can see the original walking videos from the past two years.

I originally started the walking videos in Grain Valley, Missouri. Because of the cold weather in Missouri, many days I would walk around my living room or my basement or do steps in my home just to reach a few thousand steps a day. As time went on, I needed to get more creative with the steps because I was trying to reach 10,000 steps a day...regardless if the step count was a marketing campaign or not. Some days, I felt like I needed to get out of the house no matter what. Then, I made getting out of the house and doing my walking videos a routine. Even in the winter, I was out of the house getting my walk on.

Although I didn't say so, I knew while I was doing the walking videos that my life was about to change dramatically. In the first year of the walking videos, in July 2020, I left my 12-year-long relationship, and I moved to Idaho with next to nothing. I didn't have anything. Yet, in the videos, you would never know because I only looked happy walking and being in nature. That's because when I was walking in nature, I was very happy.

I loved the trail I walked on in Missouri very much, don't get me wrong. I knew the trail so well. I knew all the turns, the shade spots, and the best places to stop and rest. I loved seeing neighbors walking beside me. The trail was only 0.9 miles, and I would make more than ten laps on the trail some days. Every time, there was something to look forward to, a new spot of shade, a new face to greet or the same old fountain for a drink of water. I can see the clear, blue Missouri sky above me, and sometimes the grey sky, too. I can still see the hill looming ahead of me in the distance, and I can still hear the neighbors' voices as they stopped and talked to me on my way home.

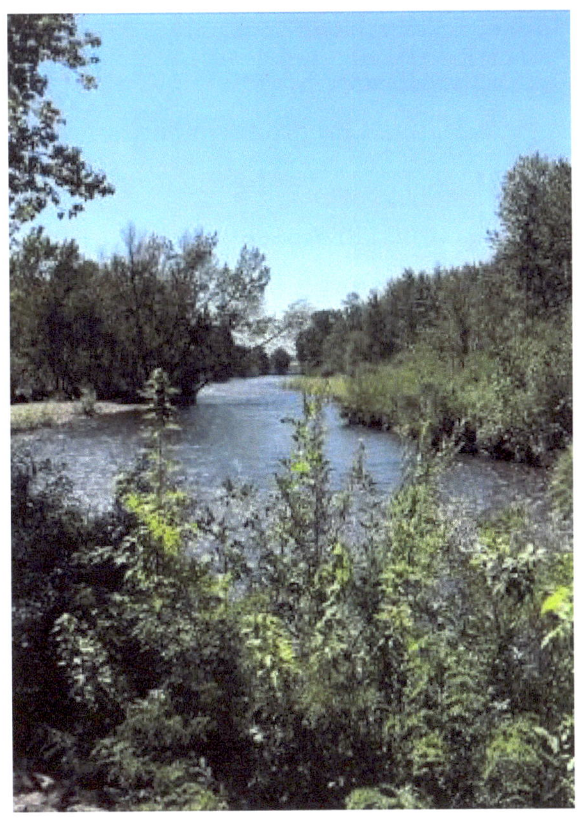

Photo by Jeanette R. Harrison, MPH

When I moved to Idaho, I felt the same kind of camaraderie on the trail that I did in Missouri. I have friends in both Missouri and Idaho that I met on the trail. Every time I go for a walk in Idaho, it's like a new adventure, and I discover something new. If I walk in a familiar place, I love seeing familiar faces. Countless times, other trail-goers and I have stopped to observe deer, beaver, birds, or other wildlife...or simply to exchange pleasantries. I love hearing the water flowing beside me in the Boise river, and I love seeing people rafting, floating, kayaking, fishing, or swimming nearby. Even if I am not on the river boating or swimming, it reminds me of times when I kayaked across and swam in lakes or played along the water's edge, whether it was a lake, river, or ocean.

Most of all, I know that whatever kind of day I'm having, if I go for a walk on the trail, I'm going to feel good when I get there and when I'm done. I know that moving my body releases hormones that make me feel better, but it's more than that. I can walk on the trail, and I feel accepted, included, a sense of belonging, and like my true self. I don't have to be anything or anyone but me when I am out walking. I can walk as long as I want (sunlight permitting), and I can walk as fast or as slow as I want. I gratefully get to spend time marveling at the trees and the ecosystems, and the amazing peacefulness that exists within a city. I'm out creating memories that I wouldn't have made in my day-to-day life, and those very memories were the ones I thought of when I had COVID myself. Those same memories also help me keep moving, from the day I wandered across a bald eagle habitat, to the day three deer were playing in the woods across the river, or to the day I noticed the beautiful archway the trees made above the trail. Every day, there is something new and special about my walk...even if that something special is making it through the heat and getting home to a nice cold glass of water.

Setting a Baseline: 2,000+ Steps

I'm an average person, just like you. I started walking a few years ago to get out of the house and to get healthier. I'm not a fitness expert, although I do have a master of public health in policy and planning. I have served in multiple administrative roles and planned dozens of programs based on current and future health policies. "Get Your Walk On" is a program I designed for myself, and I am sharing it with you.

I want to say that this book is designed for people who have an ability to walk at least 3,000 steps a day. Before beginning this or any exercise program, you should consult your healthcare provider, especially if you have any kind of health related limitations.

The content in this book is for informational, recreational, or educational purposes only and does not substitute professional medical advice or consultations with healthcare professionals.

I am not only a healthcare administrator. I also am an educator and an entrepreneur. That's the reason I created this workbook. Even the best of us need a tool to put us on the right path and to keep us going. The entrepreneurial side comes through by the creation of this workbook...

actually I will call it a walkbook. Because that is what you will be doing with this book... walking.

Before you can get started walking there are some things you will need to do first. I am going to discuss them here, and then I will give you a checklist to follow at the end of this section. At the end of each week, there will be a worksheet you can complete. You can fill it out every day or at the end of the week. There will also be a spot for you to journal about how your walking is going. I am a big fan of journaling. I believe writing about your progress allows you to reflect and improves your self-confidence. Every week you will marvel at how far you have walked and how much better you feel.

To begin with, you need to set a baseline of how much you walk every week. You can check this by wearing a fitness tracker or even checking your phone. You may also assume you walk at least 2,000 steps a day. That is how much an average person would move. That means you already probably walk one mile a day without even knowing it.

The next you need to do is to have the equipment you need to walk. I know most people think walking is putting on a pair of shoes and walking out the door. You want a pair of good quality walking and running shoes that are comfortable on your feet. You will be putting a lot of miles on these shoes, so keep in mind that shoes have a mileage, too. Generally speaking, lower cost shoes have a lower mileage because they aren't built as well. Most of my walking shoes last for about 400 miles.

You also will want a way to track all the steps you take. I use a fitness watch and my phone. I carry my phone in case my watch battery charge runs out, and then at least I have a backup. You can also use a step-counter, a pedometer, or use mile markers. One mile is about 2,000 steps for the average person.

Part of having the right equipment is wearing the right outfit. You will really be moving your body, and you will want to be comfortable while you are exercising. It is a good idea to have exercise clothes that you wear only when walking. Having the right clothing on helps you move easier and puts you in the right mindset for exercising. I often wear a hat while I am walking to cover my head from falling leaves, bugs, and to keep the sun off my scalp. I also wear sunglasses nearly every day to protect my eyes from the sun's rays. I try to use sunscreen as often as possible.

Of course, staying hydrated is essential to any exercise program. Please have a reusable water bottle or hydration pack ready to use when walking. Try not to get anything too heavy, as a heavy water bottle can lead to slouching.

I often wear earphones when I am walking to listen to music or audiobooks. You don't necessarily need earphones. You may want to listen to the sounds of nature or you may be walking with a friend while talking. However, earphones are something nice to have. Once you have all of your equipment ready to go, then you will be ready to get walking and get moving.

Get Ready to Get Your Walk On Checklist

- ☐ Consult your healthcare provider or healthcare professional to make sure a walking program is right for you.
- ☐ Have a good quality pair of walking/running shoes.
- ☐ Fitness watch, phone, step counter, pedometer, or other method to track your steps
- ☐ Exercise clothing that you will wear while walking. The clothing should be comfortable and be designated walking wear.
- ☐ Reusable water bottle or hydration pack.
- ☐ Hat or visor.
- ☐ Sunscreen.
- ☐ Earphones if you choose to listen to music or other items.
- ☐ Music playlist or audiobooks you may choose to listen to.

Week 1: 3,000 Steps

I like schedules, structures, and routine a lot. It really helps me keep my life organized and planned. I want to say here that I don't have everything planned out specifically. All the same, I do have a general schedule and plan for my day. I have included walking in that schedule. I have made walking a part of my regular routine. This week you are walking 3,000 steps a day for 5 days. That is about 30 minutes of your daily routine that you are dedicating to walking.

Usually, before I even start walking, I set a goal for how many steps I am going to take that day. This week's goal is 3,000 steps. I don't allow myself to leave the trail and head home until I have completed those 3,000 steps.

Here is how I add walking to my routine. Close to the end of every work day, I change out of my work clothes and into my walking/running clothes. I choose walking at the end of the day for two primary reasons. First, more people are on the trail at night, so I get more social interaction that way. Second, when I come home and I am tired from walking, I can eat dinner, take my bath, and relax in bed until I fall asleep. I walk in the mornings sometimes, too, so I can look at the sunrise. Find a time of day that works best for you.

While I am walking, I also have a bit of a routine. The first mile I use as a warm up. I also use it to kind of let my mind process all of the work I did earlier in the day. After I'm into my first mile, I turn on my playlist that I've labeled "Walk It Out," and I jam to my music the rest of the walk. If I've had a really hard day or have an issue I need to think about, I may just walk and listen to the sounds of the park and nature around me.

I find that having a walking routine really helps me establish goals and reach goals easier. I don't have to wonder when I am going to fit walking into my schedule because I already made it a part of my regular schedule. Hopefully, in a few weeks, it will become such a part of your schedule that you won't even have to think about it as part of your routine.

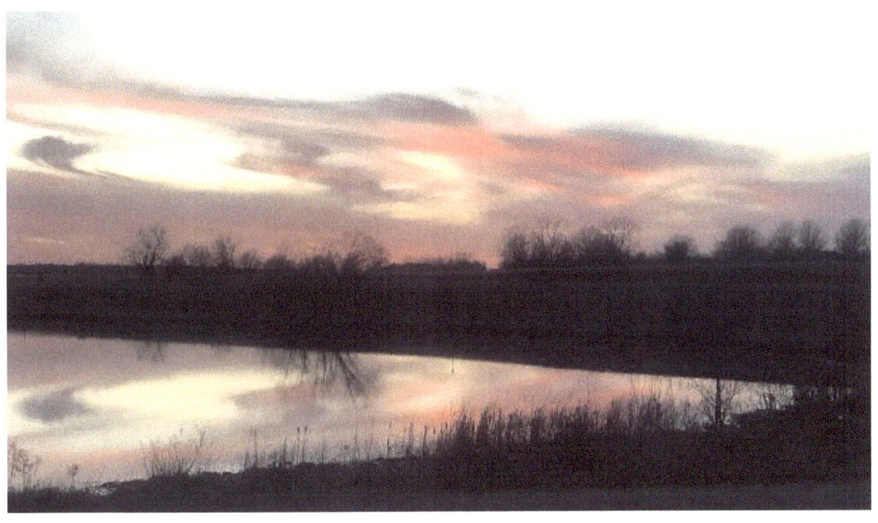

Photo by Jeanette R. Harrison, MPH

Week 1 Walking Worksheet

Days Walked	Steps	Where I Walked	When I Walked	How I Felt
Day 1				
Day 2				
Day 3				
Day 4				
Day 5				

Week 1 Walking Journal

Week 2: 4,000 Steps

It's a beautiful day today, wherever you are. Tell yourself that as you begin walking. The sun may be shining with a gentle breeze. The clouds may be rolling by with a light misting rain. Whatever the weather, it is a good day to move your body. You get to decide that it is a great day to get your walking shoes out and check out how your favorite walking trail is doing. Power up your smart watch, pull on your sneakers, fill your water bottle, and walk at your favorite trail.

You can be super happy to be walking this week because you are increasing your goal this week. This is Week 2 of Get Your Walk On, and your goal is to increase your steps this week to 4,000 steps a day. In case you are wondering, one mile is roughly 2,000 steps. Therefore, this week, your goal is to walk two miles a day for five days. Can you believe you are at two miles already!? Good for you!

I am always so glad to have the chance to cure myself of cabin fever. I hit the sidewalk, ready for the wind, ready for the sun, ready for walking. As I walk along, I wave at neighbors, smile at dogs, even bend down to pet a cat. Yes, I said it -- a cat (don't tell my dog, though). I feel something happening...this expression coming across my face by the end of the first mile. I believe it is called a smile. I am experiencing joy and happiness.

Walking has so many benefits, but one of them is that it boosts your mood. As you walk you release endorphins, and those endorphins make you feel happier. Walking also boosts your mood by relieving stress and tension. I don't know about you, but when I get home from a nice walk, I feel like all the tension in my back and shoulders has left my body.

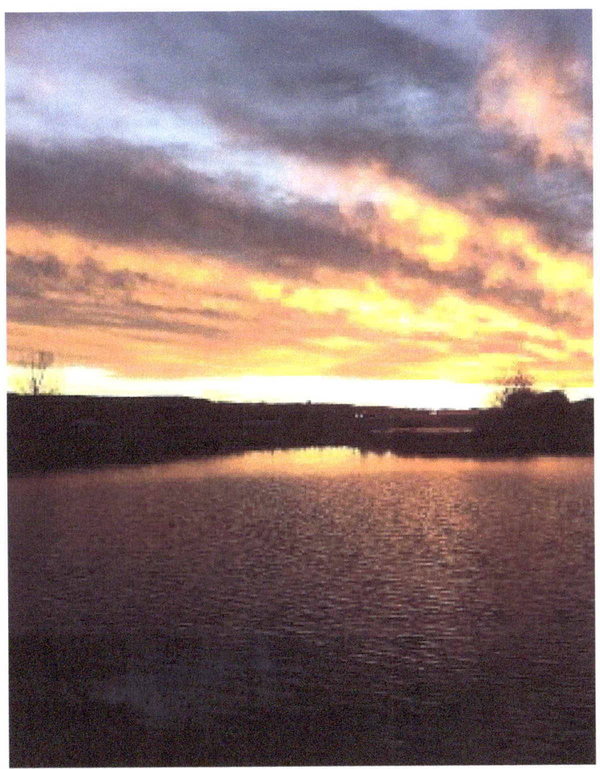

Photo by Jeanette R. Harrison, MPH

Week 2 Walking Worksheet

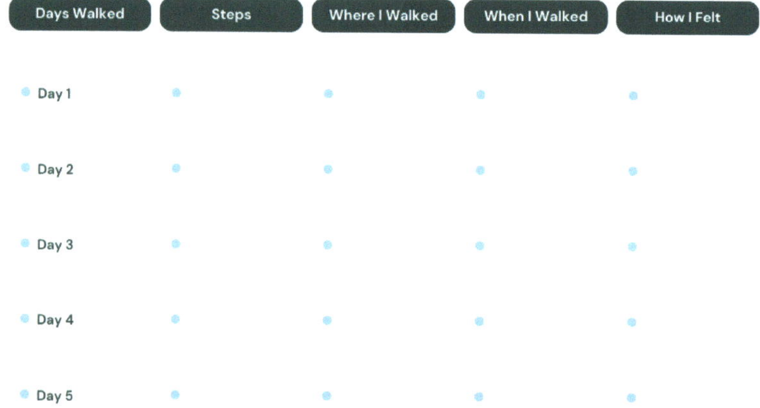

Week 2 Walking Journal

Week 3: 5,000 Steps

Congratulations! You have made it to Week 3. This week you are walking 5,000 steps a day for five days a week. That's 2.5 miles a day or 12.5 miles a week. This is a week that the transition really starts taking place. Those extra 1,000 steps a week might start to seem challenging, but you can do it!

If you are starting to feel tired, one of the reasons may be that you are not drinking enough water. On my final portion of my walk, some days I have to visualize and fantasize about what waits for me at home. I start thinking about the cool air hitting my face as I open the door, taking off my shoes and socks, and walking into the kitchen and having a big tall glass of water. Nothing is quite so refreshing as a big glass of ice water after a workout on a hot day.

I'm going to come out and admit it. I'm a big fan of water. Fill a glass up with ice cubes and some refreshing water, and I'm happy. Best drink there is. When I was a kid, I would sit down and drink my whole glass of water, and then I would fill up on another one. I would have to be reminded to eat my dinner, too.

Water doesn't only taste refreshing and feel good when you drink it, but it's good for your health, too. The human body is made up of 60% water. That's a whole lot of water going on in your body. If you are wondering where the water goes in your body, think of all those bodily fluids you have. All of those fluids need a little H2O to get going. Water doesn't only make you pee; it also helps regulate a lot of activities in your body.

If you don't get enough water, you can get dehydrated. On a hot day, dehydration can make you sick. [Signs of dehydration](#) include dark-colored urine, less frequent urination, fatigue, dizziness, confusion, diarrhea, and headaches. Drinking water during hot and humid weather replaces fluids you are losing through sweating. If you develop diarrhea from becoming dehydrated, this could cause further dehydration. Start by drinking a glass of clean, fresh drinking water if you experience any of the above symptoms.

One thing we know is that not all water is created equally. Do not drink water that has been sitting out in the sun all day, that is brown in color, or that you are unsure of the source. In those cases, be sure to plan ahead to have fresh, cool, drinking water available. Carry a water bottle with you in the summer to ensure that you have water readily available.

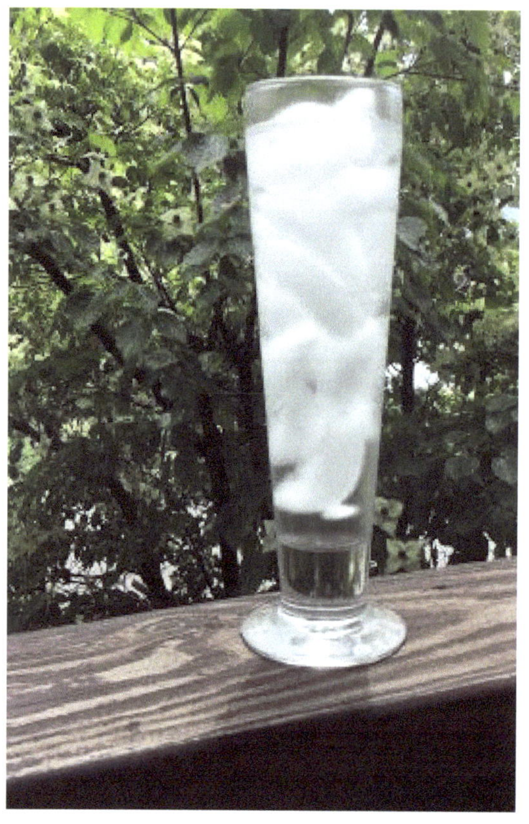

Photo by Jeanette R. Harrison, MPH

I can hear someone saying right now, "But, I don't like water. It tastes gross!" If you don't like the taste of water, maybe you can add some lemon or other fruit to the water to give it a little extra flavor. You can also try adding single-serving drink mixes.

Adding flavored packets is a nice treat, and it also gives you an added reason to drink more water during the day. One of the best things about water is that it has zero calories. Drinking that extra glass of water won't blow your diet or make you take calories away from something else. Instead of reaching for a soda or a sports drink, reach for a nice tall glass of water.

Week 3 Walking Worksheet

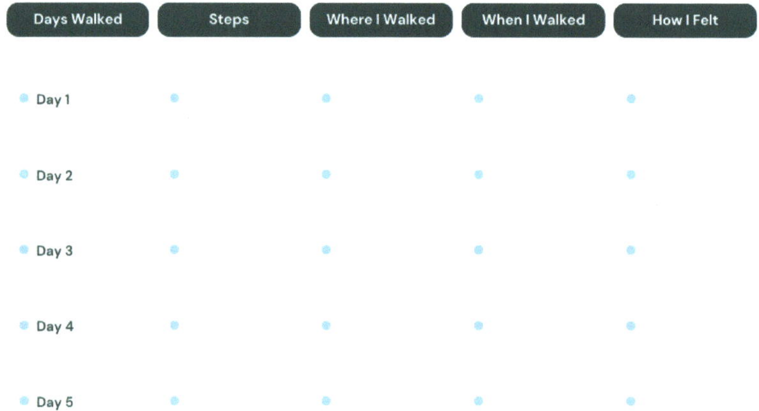

Week 3 Walking Journal

Week 4: 6,000 Steps

Can you believe you are already in Week 4? This week, you are passing the halfway point to your walking goal. You are walking 6,000 steps a day for 5 days this week. You are doing great, and now you know that you can increase your steps every week for the rest of the way. You will reach your goal of 10,000 steps a day in four more weeks!

Reaching your goals means starting your day with the right attitude. I wake up in the morning when my alarm goes off or before. I roll over, turn off the alarm, take a drink of water, say thank you for three things, and stretch as I get out of bed. My little dog stretches, too. She stretches as she begins every day. It's her way of telling me she is ready to get moving. Drinking water and stretching are important components of keeping moving.

Drinking water allows your body to function properly. Your body has something called the [sodium potassium pump](#)within the cells. Basically, the sodium potassium pump tries to keep a balance between the amount of sodium in your cells and the amount of potassium in your cells. When you get dehydrated, the cells hold onto the sodium because the cells need more

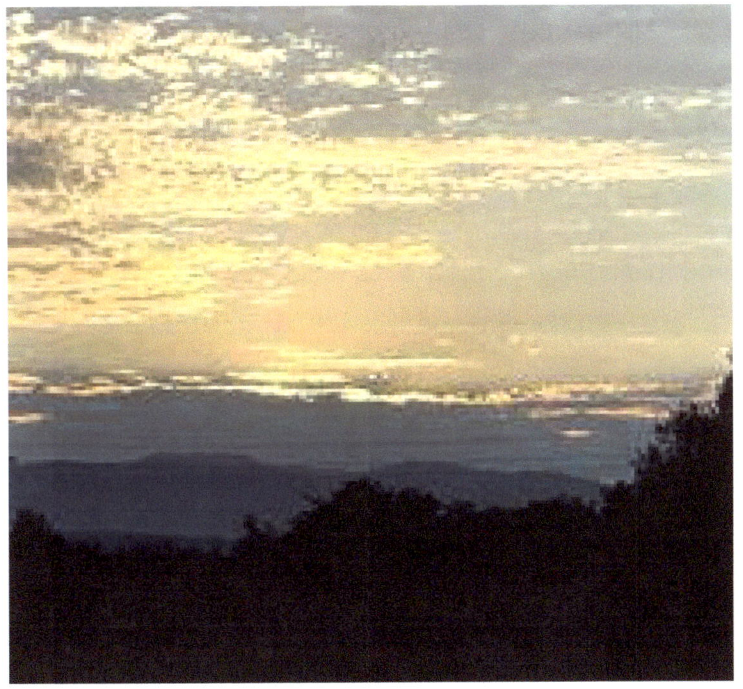

Photo by Jeanette R. Harrison, MPH

water to function. This may cause the cells to become "waterlogged" and stop working properly. Also, there is only so much space in the cells for sodium and potassium. Therefore, if you are dehydrated, the sodium is going to push the potassium out and take up space in the cell. The potassium is then passed out of the body and not used properly in the cells. A lack of potassium in the cells can lead to muscle cramping.

I remember participating in a race, and the runner in front of me knew about the sodium potassium pump, but she did not have a clear understanding of how it worked. Before the race, she had taken a sodium tablet. The sodium tablet caused her to have severe cramps, and she was forced to stop several times during the race. The sodium, along with becoming increasingly dehydrated as she was exercising, was forcing the potassium out of her cells.

No matter how hard we try, it can be hard some days to maintain the balance in the sodium potassium pump. Stretching stimulates pushing the sodium out of the cells. When I have muscle cramps, I make sure I have taken my multivitamin for the day, and I eat a banana. Bananas are high in potassium, as are other foods like oranges, raisins, prunes, apricots, potatoes, and spinach. I also make sure I do some stretches. If I start to feel a cramp on the trail, I will stop and stretch that body part. I often do my stretching after my muscles are already warm. I played tennis and soccer, and I even was a cheerleader in high school. Even back then, we knew that you had to warm up your muscles first before you stretched them or else you could sustain an injury. Stretching during the workout can also prevent an injury and help you keep moving when you are on the trail.

If you are prone to cramps during workouts, you may want to be sure to have plenty of water with you and take some potassium rich foods, like raisins, along with you. I chose raisins here because carrying a box of raisins in your pocket or a pouch takes up less space than a banana.

Week 4 Walking Worksheet

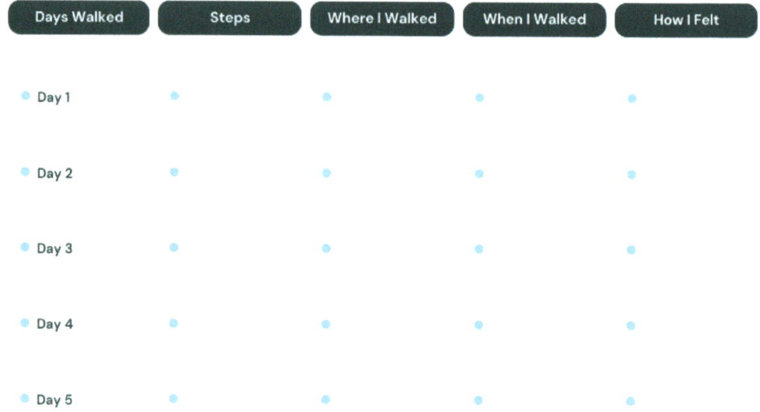

Days Walked	Steps	Where I Walked	When I Walked	How I Felt
Day 1				
Day 2				
Day 3				
Day 4				
Day 5				

Week 4 Walking Journal

Week 5: 7,000 Steps

How is your walking going? By now, you may feel like you have more energy. In fact, you should feel like you have more energy. Why? Energy creates more energy. In Week 5, you are walking 7,000 steps a day for 5 days. That's a total of 17.5 miles this week. Can you believe you have gone from walking one mile a day at your baseline to 3.5 miles a day. That's a 5K a day!

Can you notice the change in your energy? Do other people notice a change in your energy? I was asked if I have ever thought about drinking coffee with only hot water and creamer -- and leaving the actual coffee out. I smiled and told them no and assured them that I only drink one cup of coffee a day. A couple of weeks later, I had a similar conversation and the person asked how big the one cup of coffee was that I drink a day because I seemed to have "a lot of energy." I told them that I do have a lot of energy -- when I'm awake. I have always been a high-energy kind of person.

Where does my energy come from? That question can be answered by biology and physics mostly. I'm going to give you a really high-level, basic physics and biology lesson here. The law of conservation of energy says that energy is constant within a system and energy is neither created nor destroyed. That is true for the earth or the universe as a whole. There is a limited amount of energy available on the earth. However, in human beings and other [ecosystems](#), an open energy system exists. That means that the ecosystem, or the human body, in this case, has an exchange of energy inputs and outputs.

How do we input energy into our bodies? Every time we eat, we put food, or energy, into our bodies. When we count calories, we are actually counting a measurement of energy. We are counting how much energy we are putting into our bodies. Once the calories are consumed, then that food energy is converted into energy that our bodies can actually use. The energy is then used or stored in our bodies as fat cells. Fat cells are actually stored energy. Stored energy is potential energy. They contain more potential energy than other cells in your body. I was thinking the other day about how I'm not overweight – I'm full of potential energy!

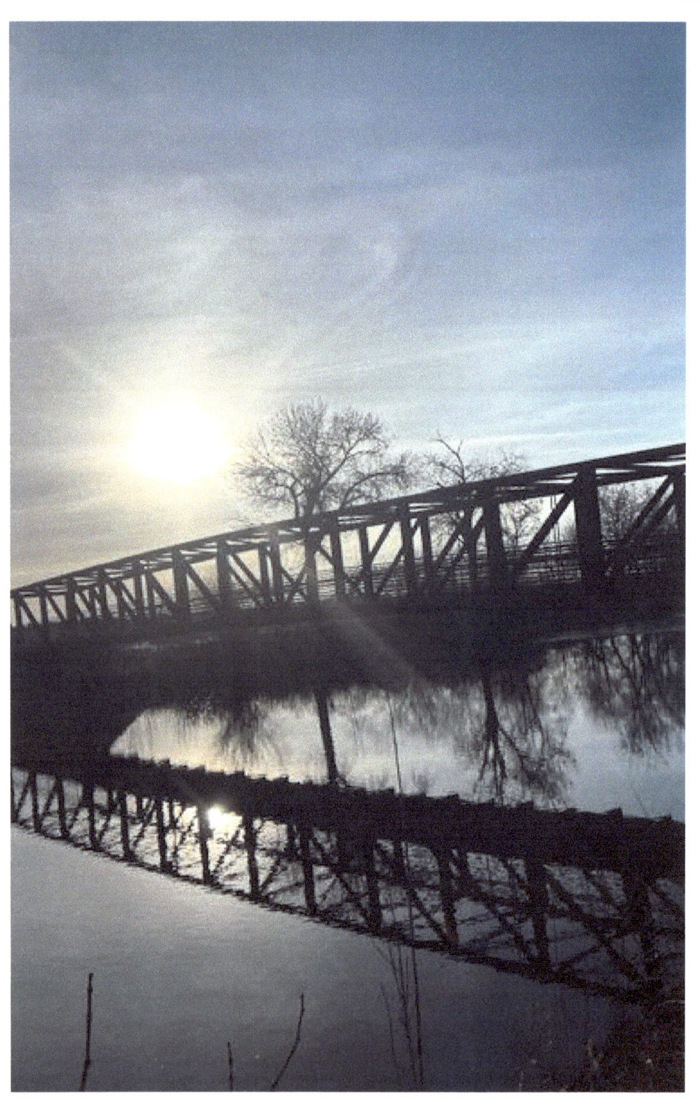

Photo by Jeanette R. Harrison, MPH

How do we input energy into our bodies? Every time we eat, we put food, or energy, into our bodies. When we count calories, we are actually counting a measurement of energy. We are counting how much energy we are putting into our bodies. Once the calories are consumed, then that food energy is converted into energy that our bodies can actually use. The energy is then used or stored in our bodies as fat cells. Fat cells are actually stored energy. Stored energy is potential energy. They contain more potential energy than other cells in your body. I was thinking the other day about how I'm not overweight, I'm full of potential energy!

How do we create energy? Newton's law of motion states that a body at rest tends to stay at rest. That is, potential energy is going to stay stored until we use it. Newton's law also states that a body in motion tends to stay in motion. When we move our bodies or exert a force, we transform that potential energy into kinetic energy. Kinetic energy is basically a body in motion. When you combine potential energy and kinetic energy, you get mechanical energy. When you exercise, you are creating mechanical energy.

POTENTIAL ENERGY + KINETIC ENERGY = MECHANICAL ENERGY

What happens when we create energy? We output energy into our environment and exchange energy with that environment.

We create force and act upon other ecosystems. We also output energy by losing weight (mass contributes to the amount of potential energy we possess), sweating, and by producing waste. The more energy we create, then the more energy we have to use. Converting potential energy into kinetic energy also triggers our brains to release hormones that make us want to create energy. When we exercise, our bodies release chemicals in the brain like norepinephrine, serotonin, dopamine, and many others. The more we exercise, the more these hormones are released and that makes us feel more energized, too.

Week 5 Walking Worksheet

Days Walked	Steps	Where I Walked	When I Walked	How I Felt
Day 1				
Day 2				
Day 3				
Day 4				
Day 5				

Week 5 Walking Journal

Week 6: 8,000 Steps

It's important to have good posture all the time, even when you are walking. When you stand up straight, shoulders back, chest out, chin up, you actually open up your airways to get the optimum level of oxygen. When you slouch, you collapse your lungs and don't let as much air in. Standing up straight strengthens your core muscles. You allow your stomach muscles to become weaker if you do not use good posture. You get tired quicker if you are slouching while walking.

This week, you are walking 8,000 steps a day. You are doing 4 miles a day and 20 miles a week. It's really important that you use every tool you have to keep going. Having good posture is one of those tools.

I practiced walking with better posture after someone took a picture of me, and I saw myself sticking my belly out and slouching while I was exercising. Oh, the horror! I vowed to do a better job of focusing on my core and walking with better posture ever since.

When you are walking, you exercise a lot of the muscles in your body. You exercise your legs, your feet (yes, your feet have muscles), your core, your back, your shoulders, your arms, and even the muscles of your neck. That is, you are exercising all of those muscles when you have good posture. When you slouch while walking or running, you don't let all the muscle groups of the body get a workout, and you don't allow the muscles to give you the maximum benefit. The more muscle groups you use when exercising, the easier the exercising becomes.

Slouching when you walk actually weakens the muscle and may contribute to back humps that can be a result of osteoporosis. Having stronger muscles in the back and legs helps strengthen your back, too. Did you know that your leg muscles actually "insert" into the lower back? If you have a low backache, you may need to stretch your legs and not just your arms and back.

Having good posture also helps with breathing, and a good breathing pattern is crucial to any workout. When you slouch or have poor posture, you collapse the respiratory system. Slouching closes up the lungs rather than opening them up and allowing more air in. It also closes up the trachea and other parts of the respiratory system. Have you ever used a hose that had a kink in it or was bent? Did you notice that the water didn't flow as freely out of the hose? That's what happens with your respiratory system when you don't have good posture. You don't allow the air to flow as freely into and out of your body. When you are exercising, your body uses more oxygen and more carbon dioxide, so you want to allow your respiratory system to work as efficiently as possible.

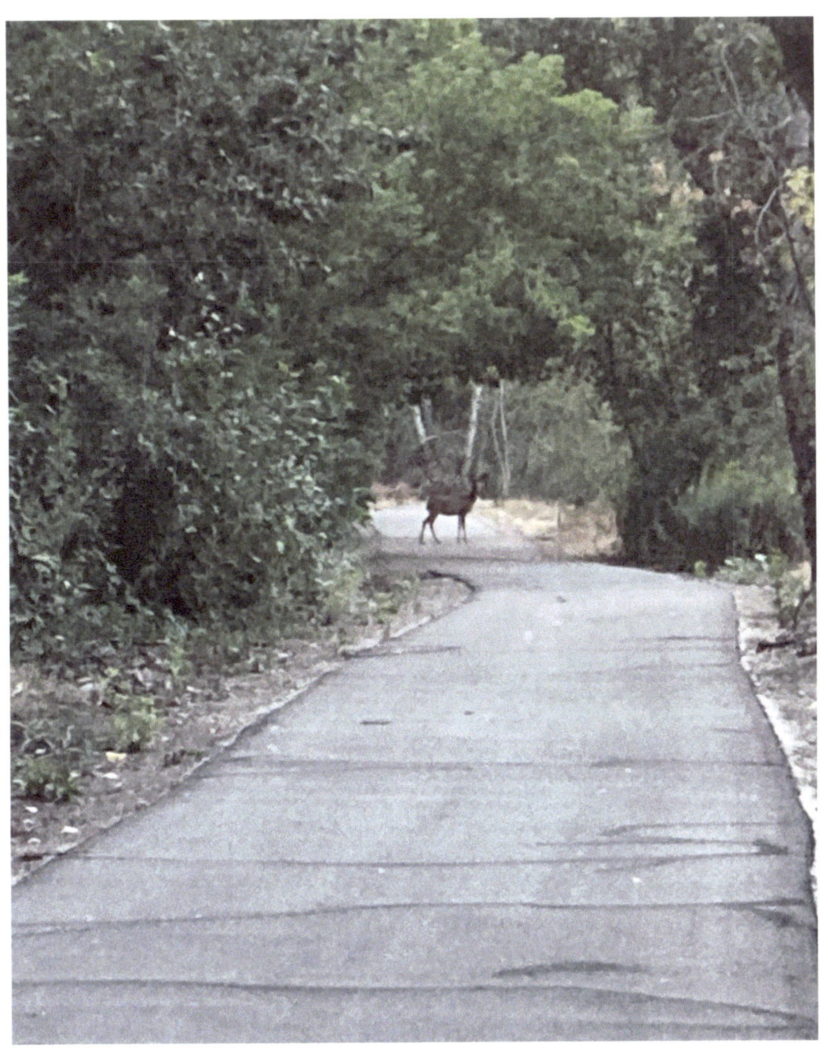

Photo by Jeanette R. Harrison, MPH

Week 6 Walking Worksheet

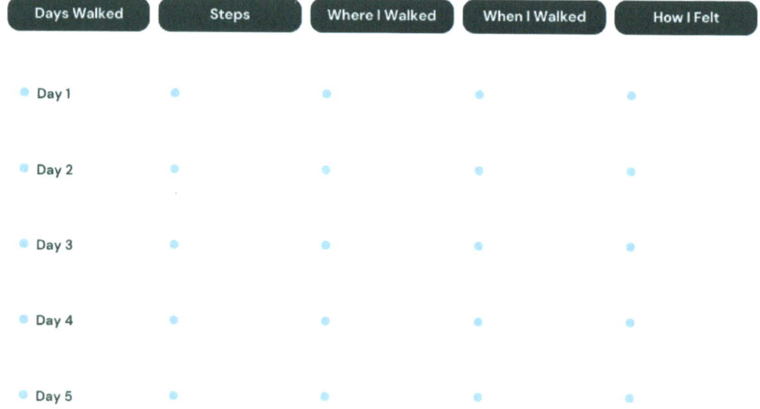

Days Walked	Steps	Where I Walked	When I Walked	How I Felt
Day 1				
Day 2				
Day 3				
Day 4				
Day 5				

Week 6 Walking Journal

Week 7: 9,000 Steps

I used to skip breakfast every day. It wasn't that I didn't like breakfast. I like breakfast a lot. I simply felt like I didn't have time, and I thought skipping that meal would help me keep my weight down. I was wrong on both counts. I credit my nurse friends who worked with me at an inner-city hospital for getting me on the eating breakfast habit. I would go into work, drop everything in my office, and they would do a pop-in. "Hey, I noticed your door was open. Do you want to go grab some breakfast with me?" I said I would go with them, but I really didn't eat breakfast. "Oh, you have to eat breakfast," they told me. Fortunately, the hospital where I worked had a terrific breakfast spread in the cafeteria, so I was hooked. I still make myself breakfast -- even if it's some fruit and cereal -- every day.

This week, you are walking 9,000 steps. That is 4.5 miles a day. Walking 4.5 miles a day takes a lot of energy. I discussed how eating provides fuel for your body. I'm going to give a really short biology lesson about how food is converted into energy. Our bodies use glucose to create energy and keep our bodies moving. When your body creates energy, molecules first must go through the cellular respiration cycle. Simple and complex carbohydrates are recognized in the part of the cycle known as glycolysis. Proteins contain amino acids and enter cellular respiration at the intermediate stage and go through the citric acid cycle and electron transport. Fats contain triglyceride molecules that can be used in the glycolysis phase and also molecules that are used in the citric acid cycle. Insulin allows the cells to absorb glucose which provides energy to the cells. When you eat breakfast, you allow this process to start every morning. You are telling your body that you are ready for it to start producing energy and start working for the day.

Because eating breakfast tells your body to start producing insulin every day, it also can reduce your risk of diabetes. Eating breakfast helps regulate your body's blood sugar levels and prevents blood sugar spikes throughout the day. Individuals over the age of 40 are at higher risk of diabetes. Multiple studies have also shown that eating breakfast reduces the risk of heart disease and atherosclerotic disease. A study from the University of Iowa College of Public Health published in the Journal of the American College of Cardiology, found that people who did not eat breakfast had an 87% higher risk of death from cardiovascular disease. The reasons behind this are not entirely clear at this point. However, eating breakfast helps regulate cholesterol, insulin, and satiety (aka hunger) throughout the day. These factors all can contribute to healthier cardiovascular functioning.

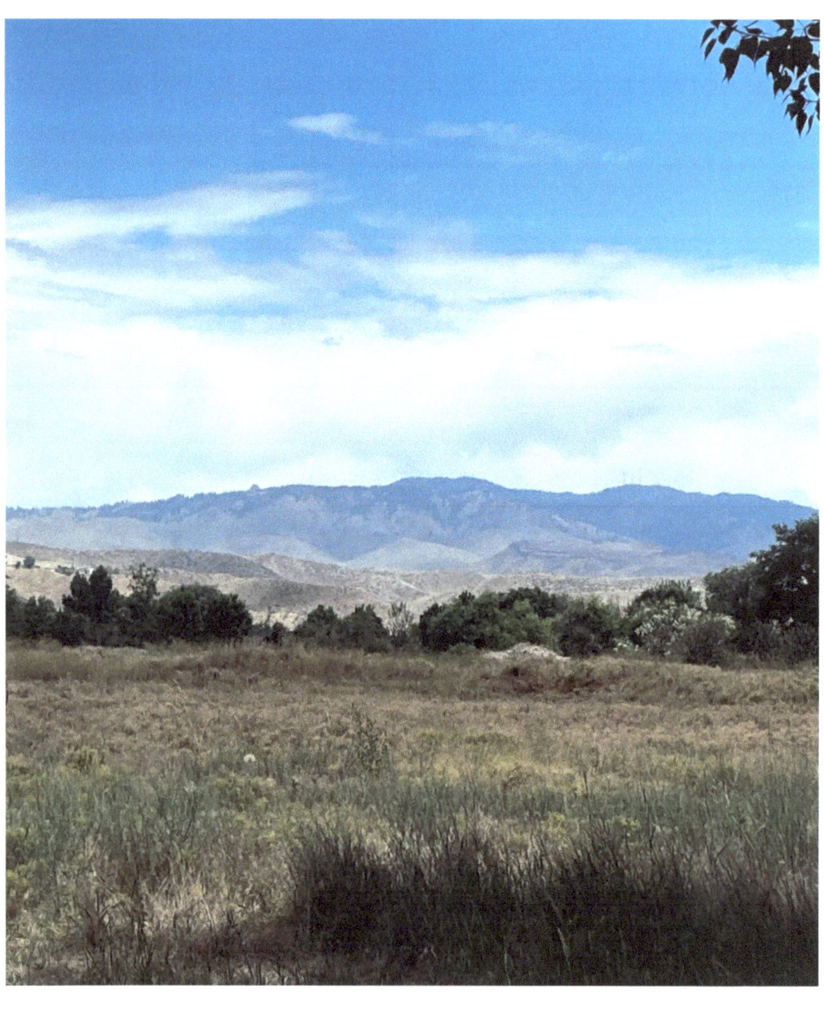

Photo by Jeanette R. Harrison, MPH

Week 7 Walking Worksheet

Days Walked	Steps	Where I Walked	When I Walked	How I Felt
Day 1				
Day 2				
Day 3				
Day 4				
Day 5				

Week 7 Walking Journal

Week 8: 10,000 Steps

You have officially made it to the last week of the program! Congratulations! You are probably feeling all kinds of emotions – relief, joy, empowerment, exhaustion, fulfillment. You may be celebrating yourself and you may feel like crying, too. Why do you feel like crying, though? Exercising provides an emotional release.

A few years ago, I had been out walking several miles one day after work. It was a beautiful evening, the sun was shining, and the walkers were friendly. Everything seemed picture perfect. Then, as I walked into the door of my home, I started crying. I wondered to myself, "Why on earth am I crying? What is this about? I just had a great day."

I did, in fact, have a great day. I liked my job at the time, I felt like I was making a difference in the world, I had things to do, places to go, people to see. I also under the surface was upset about so many things. The tears that day weren't about my day, or even about that week, or especially about that walk...they were an emotional release I felt after having exercised. Exercise often can be an emotional release because the energy we usually use to keep it all together, we have used up in our exercise routine. Then, we are amazingly able to let go of pent up frustrations, hurts, feelings, stress...and let it all out.

I also use exercise, walking especially, as a time to go over things in my mind. For some reason, I find that skipping to my favorite tunes and having the wind blow in my hair and the sun on my face, gives me a sense of clarity I can't get anywhere else. I can think about all of the things in life that I didn't have time to deal with at the moment, or that I wanted to reevaluate. Almost as soon as I get home, I see things so much more clearly. It's amazing.

For me, and for many people, exercise provides a great way to sort out my thoughts and even to make plans for my life. I've written more than one article, post, presentation, paper, and even chapters in a book in my head while I was walking. I'm glad I can do that, because writing, too, is a release to me. It's a way that I can get my thoughts out. I once had someone ask, how do you write in your truest voice? I write in the voice as if no one is reading. I write in the voice I think to myself as I am walking all alone on the trail, and it is just the wind and the trees and the trail and grass and distant traffic. That is how I write in my truest voice. That is how I gain clarity and release when I am walking and writing.

To me, walking is a great problem solver. I suddenly see things as they were...the friend who was incredibly kind and gracious, why a meeting went better than I had planned, how my day was actually super amazing, how I really do feel 27 still (even though I'm not 27), and how I really have had so many tremendous awesome experiences in my life that no one can take from me. It's a great feeling.

The best release, though, that I get from walking is the sense of accomplishment I have when I get home. This week, you are walking 10,000 steps a day. At the end of every walk, give yourself a fist pump in the air! You are doing this for you. You should be so proud of what you have accomplished. You walked because it was something you wanted for yourself. You set a goal and reached that goal because you wanted to. Good for you!

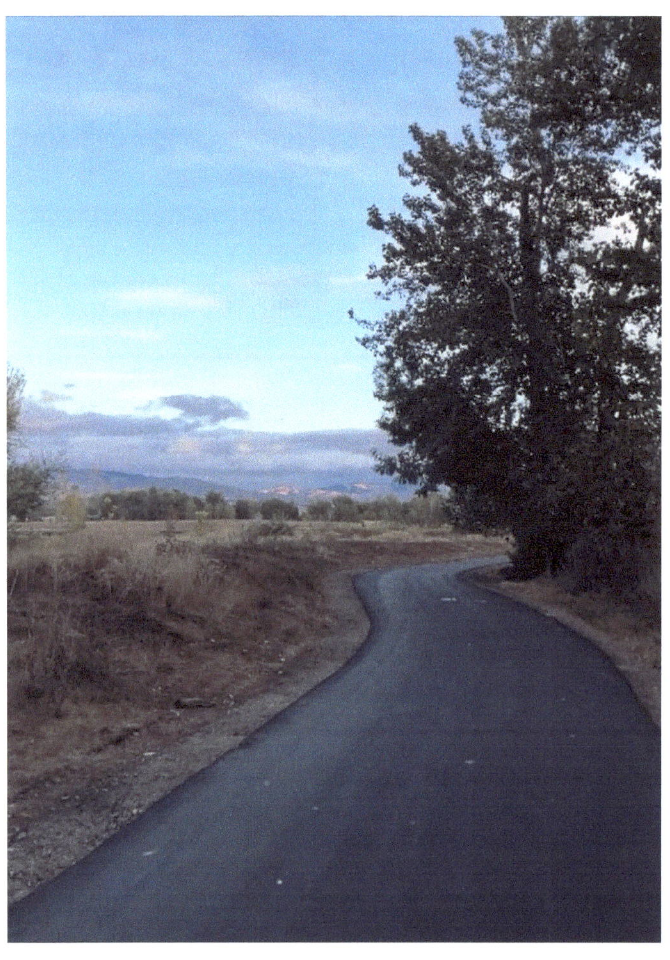

Photo by Jeanette R. Harrison, MPH

Week 8 Walking Worksheet

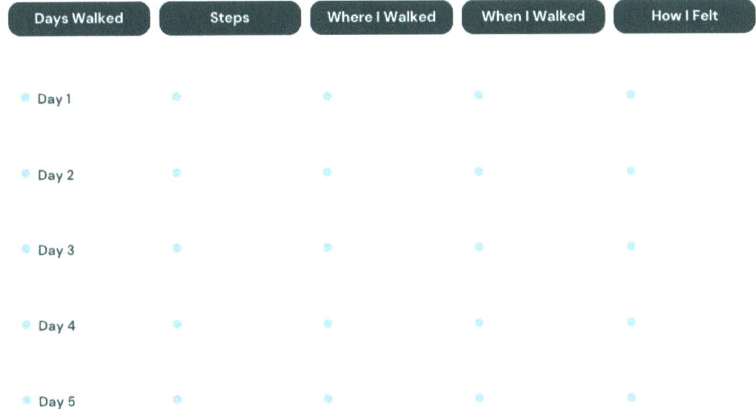

Days Walked	Steps	Where I Walked	When I Walked	How I Felt
Day 1				
Day 2				
Day 3				
Day 4				
Day 5				

Week 8 Walking Journal

Keep Walking, Keep Moving

Now that you have reached 10,000 steps a day, the real challenge begins. That challenge is to keep on walking. Over the past several months, you have walked in the cold, in the rain, in the sunshine, in the wind. You have walked in living rooms, basements, gyms, on sidewalks, trails, and maybe some treadmills. I don't know about anyone else, but I wore out at least one pair of shoes over the past 8 weeks.

For some sports and activities, once the season is over, the participants take a breather and wait until next season starts. They take a break. That's the amazing thing about walking. You don't have to take a break. You can keep going right from where you are today. I know that I am planning on going for a walk this afternoon. It should be about a 5 miles walk, and I set a goal to walk 7 miles a day five days a week by the end of this month.

Of course, walking, like any kind of exercise, takes time and commitment. As a result, I plan accordingly. I know that I can walk in the afternoons, come home, eat dinner, take a hot bath, read a book, do some light work, watch TV, or whatever helps me relax. By making walking and the activities associated with it enjoyable, it motivates me to want to get up and do the whole thing all over again the next day.

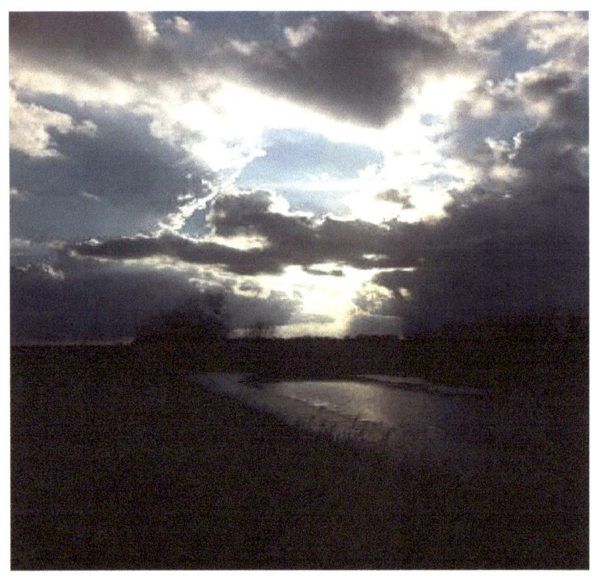

Photo by Jeanette R. Harrison, MPH

Now that you have reached your 10,000 steps a day, it is time to set a new goal. You may want to participate in a 5K or 10K race, play tennis, golf, go hiking, or start cycling. Hopefully, this walking program has helped you see that you can do it... no matter what you choose. I'm so glad you chose to get your walk on!

Acknowledgements

I would like to express my gratitude to my countless friends and family who supported me in my own walking journey. They spent hours watching videos, reading blog posts, and supporting my efforts.

I am deeply grateful for the American Public Health Association and the Keep It Moving campaign. This campaign empowered me to put my shoes on and get walking several years ago. Based on my own walking experiences, I was able to put together this book.

I would finally like to thank the communities where I live for having a commitment to outdoor pathways that are safe and accessible to all to use in a public place. An ability to exercise on prebuilt pathways was essential to being able to get my own walk on.

About the Author

Jeanette R. Harrison, MPH, has over 25 years experience in healthcare and education. She has served as a healthcare administrator, faculty member, and is currently the owner and CEO of How Healthcare Works, LLC.

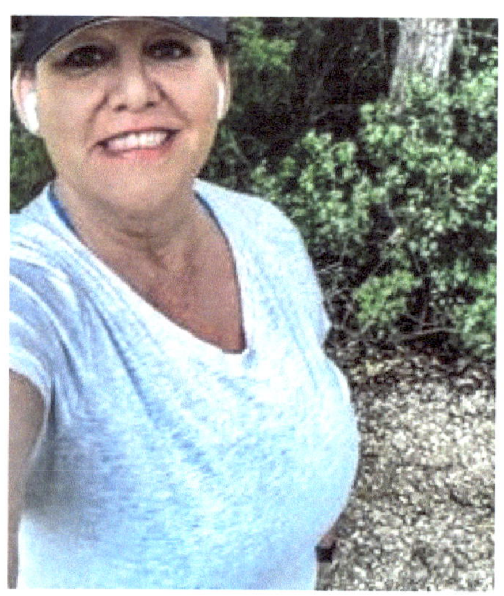